ADULT DYSLEXIA

TIPS AND TRICKS FOR BEATING IT

ANTHONY EKANEM

Contents

Preface

Dyslexia is a learning disorder that affects an individual's ability to read, spell, write, or speak. Those who have it are often very smart and hardworking, but they have difficulty connecting the alphabets they see to the sounds those alphabets represent. Dyslexia affects mainly the areas of the brain that process language.

Dyslexia is an inherent weakness in short-term memory that is either auditory or visual. It can make it extremely difficult for a person to learn and understand the relation between symbols and spoken sounds. This difficulty makes the person unable to correctly pronounce words in such a way that makes a word or sentence sound proper.

The severity of the problem of adult dyslexia varies widely among dyslexic people. The main areas of difficulty include reading, writing, spelling, numeric, personal organisation and time-keeping. However, the degree to which it affects individuals may be from mild spelling difficulties to severe organisational problems or complete illiteracy. In all reality, there is nothing like a typical case of dyslexia.

In most cases, people with dyslexia are unaware that they are suffering from such a problem. In contrast, others have not had a confirmed diagnosis until adulthood. Adult dyslexia can be difficult to recognise and identify as it is a problem that many people do not realise they have, or they try to hide it. Simple tasks that an individual with dyslexia may perform may become increasingly difficult, such as taking down a message, and this can lead to frustration and anxiety.

What Causes Adult Dyslexia

Most research has concentrated on explaining the causes of dyslexia. This has, however, proved to be rather unsuccessful. Neurological research suggests there may be an abnormality in the functioning of the left side of the brain that controls the speech system. Cognitive research, on the other hand, has increasingly focused on problems of phonological awareness (the awareness of the speech sounds within words). There have been speculations that these problems may be associated with a specific area of the brain.

One thing is conclusive, however, and that is the fact that the causes of dyslexia centre around an abnormality in the brain which prevents an individual from correctly recognising the right speech pattern. Many people that do not have dyslexia can also switch sounds out of their correct pattern. This suggests to researchers that perhaps it is something that can be corrected in everyone.

Whatever the cause dyslexia may be, there is no doubt that dyslexia leads to many literacy problems in individuals. It also leads to insensitivity to sounds within a word. In time, this will lead to problems with reading as well as reading comprehension. The causes of dyslexia can vary from person to person, and this can make treatment a bit difficult.

Estimates of the number of dyslexic people vary immensely – from four per cent to ten per cent of the population. It is believed to be about four times more prevalent in males than females. Statistics in this area have been difficult to gather with accuracy due to people not willing to admit to having a dyslexic problem.

What Are The Symptoms Of Adult Dyslexia?

Dyslexia can present itself in many ways, and it is more than likely that all the following symptoms will not present themselves in one individual. However, use this to see which ones may apply to you.

- A difference between the individual's academic performance and real-life achievements in practical problem-solving and verbal skills

- Taking an excessive amount of time to read a book and finish it

- Missing the endings of words in reading and spelling

- A poor presentation of written work, such as poor spelling and use of punctuation

- Inability to think what to write

- Reluctance in writing things down, including messages

- Confusing telephone messages

- Difficulty in note-taking

- Difficulty in following what others say

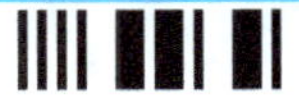

- Difficulty with verbal patterns

- Time management problem

- Leaving words out

- Difficulty remembering tables

- Difficulty with mental mathematics

Again, all these symptoms may not present themselves typically within one individual. However, if any of the symptoms applies to you, consult your doctor for a possible diagnosis.

CHAPTER ONE

The Strengths Dyslexic People Have

Despite the difficulties caused by dyslexia, many dyslexic people have risen to prominence in their specialised fields. Albert Einstein and Leonardo da Vinci probably had dyslexia based on reports and the information available. Jackie Stewart and Susan Hampshire are two highly successful people who had dyslexia.

Dyslexic people are often very good at visually-based skills such as art, sculpture, design, architecture and engineering. Naturally, we see people that have diminished verbal or language skills or ability, have a higher plain of logic and reasoning. They are often very creative and original thinkers that can succeed at very high levels of endeavour. Often, they may offer their unusual way of solving problems. Because having dyslexia may provoke them to succeed, they usually have a high degree of determination that help them in many other facets of their life or career.

With all the negative attention that surrounds dyslexia, numerous people have overcome the challenge and risen to prominent positions in their respective fields. There is no reason why you should be different. All it takes is the desire and will to succeed, and the effort and patience needed to get it done.

CHAPTER TWO

How Do You Know You Have Dyslexia?

Whether at work or school, the best way to determine whether you have dyslexia or not is to obtain an assessment or test from your doctor. Here are some reasons to get tested and the benefits of an assessment:

- It can reveal difficulties which can be overcome with proper training.

- It may help clarify the reasons behind the difficulties with written work so that appropriate measures can be taken.

- It puts any difficulties into perspective and identifies areas of strength you may have.

- It can help admissions tutors or potential employers to judge a person's suitability for a particular course or job.

- It can help to secure additional grants to pay for extra training or equipment which might be needed.

- It may reveal that extra time would be needed for some examinations to compensate for being dyslexic.

There are two types of dyslexia tests available. These are screening tests and comprehensive tests.

SCREENING TESTS

These type of tests are designed to be used on many people, to narrow down the group to who might need a more thorough examination for possible dyslexia. The purpose is to ensure that anyone who does not meet specific criteria is not tested over and again. The tests are not for dyslexia. Instead, they are designed to help researchers focus on people who have difficulties with their studies, work or other activities and who might have dyslexia.

Typically, these tests consist of a shortlist of questions, such as:

1. Do you have difficulties with spelling?
2. Do you find directions confusing?
3. Were you reluctant to go to school?
4. Do you have problems with mathematics?

Students, in particular, selected by this method, could be having problems with learning for any number of reasons. These could be emotional problems, Attention Deficit (ADHD), delayed learning, autism, dysphasia, and possible dyslexia. Screening tests like these cannot be regarded as valid tests for dyslexia, but they are beneficial for researchers. Dyslexia is still in a state where vast amounts of research are still needed to fully understand what causes it and what the most effective treatments for it are.

COMPREHENSIVE TESTS

A comprehensive test for dyslexia looks at the whole person and examines the root cause of any learning difficulties. The word 'comprehensive' means 'thorough', and these tests examine which brain functions are interfering with a person's acquisition of normal learning. Tests of reading, spelling, comprehension, and intelligence are given, as well as visual tests, visual scanning tests, sequencing, reversals and other tests of such a nature.

A comprehensive dyslexia test may be administered in two ways, either by a psychologist or at a distance. It is not yet known which method is most effective to determine the best test available, as such a thing will vary from person to person and depends on the case.

Comprehensive testing by a psychologist

Psychologists operate either through schools and colleges or privately in a consulting room. Some higher institutions have psychologists available. If you are a student at that institution, such resources may be available to you. If you know any psychologist in your school, contact them to find out about getting an assessment. For those who are no longer in school, many well-qualified psychologists are available to offer such services.

Assessment by a psychologist - if one is available - seems to be the method that works for the majority of people living with dyslexia. However, like with anything else, there are a fair number of people who are dissatisfied with the process. Some people have reported that some psychologist denied that dyslexia existed. Again, finding the right one for you takes a little time and research.

Some people seek an individual assessment by a psychologist. Although expensive, this is more straightforward. Many people have reported having paid a lot of money for a private assessment, but the costs vary from one country to another, and from facility to another. The assessment takes a few hours, and you should expect to receive a detailed report. Although assessments are thorough, few psychologists provide detailed recommendations for improving a person's learning techniques.

COMPREHENSIVE TESTING AT A DISTANCE

An alternative is comprehensive dyslexia testing at a distance. This has the advantage of improved objectivity. The psychologist remains utterly objective about the person's performance in all the tests, as he or she never meets the person, but bases the assessment mainly on the test results. This, in a scientific sense, is the most successful of the tests available.

The tests used are very similar to those used by psychologists in schools or privately, but have been adapted so that adults at home can use them. This type of test produces more detailed assessment report than a psychologist in school typically provides. It contains detailed recommendations for learning techniques that will help the person raise their achievement level.

CHAPTER THREE

Where Can You Be Assessed?

There are centres and institutions where you can have an assessment by an independent, professionally qualified psychologist who has specialist knowledge of dyslexia. It is helpful for the psychologist to have background information from employers or tutors. However, sometimes people wish to obtain advice before involving anyone else. The Consulting Psychologists will, of course, treat confidentially all information received and will not release any information without the permission of the person concerned.

The assessment lasts about two hours, which includes time to discuss the findings and talk about ways of approaching any difficulties which may have been revealed. It will investigate the individual's thinking, learning, and problem-solving skills to obtain indications of areas of strength and difficulty. It will also examine attainments in the necessary skills of reading, writing, spelling and mathematics.

With the results, the psychologist will then assess whether there are areas where performance is not up to the expected level. When this is the case, it is often a sign that a specific learning difficulty exists, which has made it particularly hard to develop specific skills. Further testing and discussion will have explored possible reasons for this.

WHAT HELP IS AVAILABLE?

Following the assessment session, the psychologist will give practical advice according to the severity of any difficulties and the educational and career goals being sought. Typically, advice and recommendations include:

1   Making others aware of the presence of dyslexia so that they do not always criticise poor spelling or handwriting

2. A recommendation that extra time be allowed or other special arrangements made so that specific difficulties do not unduly affect performance in examinations

3. Provision of computer support to minimise the impact of specific spelling difficulties

4. A short course designed to improve performance in some or all the following skills: spelling, report-writing, study-skills, revision and exam techniques, time-management and general organisation

5. An individualised learning programme designed to address deficiencies in necessary skills.

CHAPTER FOUR

Is Specialist Tuition Available?

Remedial provision will, of course, depend on the severity of the difficulties experienced. Adult dyslexics may well have acquired strategies to improve reading fluency and speed, and they may make greater use of diagrams and illustrations. Writing and spelling difficulties may require a sustained period of specialist teaching, but most problems are not insuperable. Many adults quickly gain confidence as they receive help.

Training programmes have several essential components:

- To accommodate weaknesses in short-term memory; material to be learned must be made more manageable.

- To compensate for perceptual weakness, a multi-sensory method of teaching is adopted, which stimulates learning by using all the senses.

- Mnemonics, visual images, mind maps, speed reading and other techniques may be used.

CAN MODERN TECHNOLOGY HELP?

There are many devices which are now available, which can be of practical help, but much will depend on the nature and extent of the individual's disability. These include:

1. **Spell-checkers and grammar checkers**. Most modern computers have a spell-check function which many dyslexic people find invaluable. Some also have a grammar checker.

2. **Electronic dictionaries.** These offer the meaning of words or alternatives and are quicker to use than conventional dictionaries.

3. **Dictating machines and tape recorders.** If audio-typing facilities are available, these can be invaluable.

4. **Calculators.** Even a simple calculator can be a blessing for someone who has difficulty with numbers

5. **Memory telephones.** Telephones that can store and automatically dial pre-entered numbers may be useful.

6. **Electronic schedulers.** These can be used as a reminder for appointments, meetings or remembering essential tasks.

7. **Voice-activated computers.**These allow full control through the voice, including dictating to the word-processor. They are, however, costly.

8. **Tinted glasses and coloured overlays.**Some people find these useful.

CHAPTER FIVE

Compassion for People with Dyslexia

Dyslexia is a disability and people must comply with the Disability Discrimination Act of 1995. Here are some tips for those you may know that are dyslexic or those you wish to become more understanding of the issue:

1 Be supportive, show understanding and give encouragement when appropriate

2 Don't regard dyslexic people as a 'problem.'

3. Concentrate on their strengths and don't force them to do things against their will

4. Try to tailor the job to suit the person

5. Be aware that some dyslexic people may appear to be very confident, to cover up the stress which they may be experiencing

6. If the dyslexic colleague wishes it, recommend an assessment by an educational psychologist

7 Circulate information well in advance of meetings to allow plenty of time for it to be assimilated

8 Print text on pale-coloured papers

9. Help with checking text if asked to do so

10. Highlight important text when circulating documents

11. Make verbal instructions brief and clear

12. Use multi-sensory aids on training courses.

CHAPTER SIX

How Can You Afford the Available Help?

The funding of dyslexia assessment and tuition for adults can be difficult, and to many dyslexic adults, this can be an insurmountable hurdle. In some countries, local education authorities sometimes run basic skills courses free of charge. However, these courses are not targeted at people who have dyslexia or taught by teachers who have a dyslexia qualification. The cost of assessment and an ongoing teaching programme can be quite high. Many adults sometimes seek help to meet these costs. You can obtain help from any of the following:

1. If you are a full-time student, you may be eligible for a Disabled Student's Allowance (available in some countries), which you can use to buy items such as specialist equipment or essential texts, or specialist help. Your Disabled Students Advisor should be able to help you with this.

2. Some employers partly or wholly fund assessments and lessons

3. If you are unemployed, you can contact the Department for Education and Employment's Disability Employment Advisor (if this is available in your locality). You can be referred for assessment by a Placement, Assessment and Counseling Team which has contracts with the Dyslexia Institute and may fund lessons.

4. Unemployed adults may also seek work under the New Deal Scheme. As part of this, it may be possible to receive specialist tuition.

5. A local charitable organisation may be able to help.

6. The Dyslexia Institute provides funds for a small number of bursaries each year.

CHAPTER SEVEN

Tips to Help with Adult Dyslexia

The following are some helpful tips and tricks for you to try to cope with and hopefully beat dyslexia:

1. **Instead of visualising words, try to make them more concrete to stand out.**

One of the powerful ways for those that have difficulty with particular words is to make the process of understanding the word and its sounds less visual and more concrete. Sometimes even just writing them on paper does not also work. In those cases, get creative. Write it down on a chalkboard or use colour forms. This can be effective in allowing your mind to wrap itself around the word in a more contextualised way.

2. **Build your confidence in any way you deem fit.**

This is another easy and effective way to help you overcome dyslexia. Many times, frustrations and stress can compound the situation. When you feel that way, start to focus on some of the things that you are great at, and you excel. Sometimes, even the smallest boost of confidence can do wonders.

3. **Read out loud whenever you can.**

Another good one to try. Sometimes the situation does not warrant you to be able to read aloud but whenever you get the chance to, go for it. Areas of the brain tend to remember this type of action.

4. Make a mental picture as much as you can.

We talked earlier about trying to visualise less and make things more concrete; now try the opposite approach if the specific way is not working for you. Dyslexia has no common cases, and difficulties vary from person to person. With some, it does help to visualise a word as you saw it spelt correctly.

5. Mnemonic spelling can be an excellent tool to use.

This one takes a detailed oriented person to use, but it can be done. If you are good with Mnemonic devices, then try this with words you have difficulty spelling. Such as BECAUSE: Big Elephants Can't Always Use Small Elevators. Or Friend: Every friend has an I, and hopefully it will never END. Get creative.

Here is a list of other Mnemonic devices for words that are commonly difficult among people with dyslexia:

- **Because**- Bake Every Cake And Use Six Eggs.
- **Said** - Sally Ann Is Dancing
- **Could**- Can Oliver Understand Long Division
- **Rhythm**- Rhythm Has Your Two Hips Moving
- **They**- They Hate Eating Yogurt
- **Wednesday**- WE Do Not Eat Sweets DAY
- **Tuesday**- U Eat Sweets DAY
- **Again**- Again, Gorillas Appear In Nighties

1. Start trying to learn the phonetics and rules of spelling and grammar logically.

2. Set up extra time to complete work or examinations whenever possible to ensure that stress does not set in from not having enough time.

3. Repeat instructions or directions to yourself as much as you can, and as soon as you are given them. This will help you to remember them accurately.

4   Do whatever you can to block out unneeded noise, this can disrupt proper thought and concentration.

5   If you are a student, then sit in front of the class so that others around you are not distracting.

6   Use a computer as often as you can. This allows for greater ease at seeing any mistakes you may make and less second-guessing on your part.

With a little adjustment in learning strategies, even a person affected by adult dyslexia can improve their reading and writing skills. You need to understand that every human being is different. Different brains are wired differently. You cannot expect everyone to be an expert in one field. Some students are good at Mathematics, while others are good at literature or other subjects.

Even if a person is affected by adult dyslexia, it can mean that they will be weak learners in just one aspect, that is, reading or writing. From no angle would it mean that they are dumb and worthless. They may be good and highly talented in some other fields that do not involve reading and writing, such as painting.

The adjustment in learning strategies must be made based on the unique talent that the person possesses. Thus, the first task is to study the person and identify their strengths.

Feelings of rejection are normal with dyslexia. In general, a person with dyslexia does not get a good response from their surroundings. People at school, in their neighbourhood, and even immediate family, often start to taunt them or ridicule them, considering them to be dumb and stupid. Such behaviour can have a severe impact on their self-confidence, causing feelings of isolation and rejection.

Therefore, once the problem is identified, through a dyslexia test, proper actions must be taken, showing that they have the talent to achieve success. It can be difficult to win self-confidence back, but that is why this is the stage that must be won before coping is possible.

One way to improve the reading and writing skills of someone who has dyslexia is by focusing on building the phonetic decoding skills. Since dyslexia causes slower reading, teaching to break words into their basic sounds and then rearrange these sounds to produce different words is very beneficial.

Such training will gradually help an adult with dyslexia learn to read more accurately and at a higher speed.

CHAPTER EIGHT

Tips to Help Remember Numbers

Counting out change. If you are slow in counting out change, that can be embarrassing. A method of dealing with this is that you should always have available a bill more extensive than the estimated amount of the sale. This way, you get a lot of change accumulating. Get rid of this change by counting out the exact amount of small purchase that you know the precise amount of and putting it into a change purse. When you buy your morning coffee, the seller may wonder why you always have the correct amount every time. The above may seem trivial, but it is crucial, and it protects your self-esteem.

Difficulty in mathematics. Visualising a pattern of the appropriate number of dots around a number allows you to count them and thereby solve the problem. You can also remember the pattern of the dots on a dice to help, for example, six is two rows of three, and five is a square of four with one more in the centre.

Phone Numbers. When you cannot remember a phone number long enough to walk across the room and dial it, try "drawing on the right side of the brain". It teaches the right-brain or left-brain usage to "normal" people. However, for some, it teaches them how to organise and separate the right and left brain's functioning for the first time. Now, with concentration, you can remember a phone number for a minute or so.

Dealing with numbers. When dealing with numbers, like balancing your chequebook or paying bills, read the number backward (from right to left) to yourself and then write it. To check yourself, read the number you wrote the other direction and check it against the original. You will find that if you break up the repetitive pattern, you recognise mistakes better.

Number 7. If your '7's look like '1's, put a line through the downstroke and then there is no way it can be mistaken for a '1'.

Remembering numbers. When remembering numbers, like phone numbers, try saying the first three numbers as a whole number, and the last four digits as two whole numbers. Example 827-1456: Eight hundred and twenty-seven, fourteen fifty-six. This allows you to visualise the sounds of the words and makes it harder to forget them.

Try remembering your PIN-code and some telephone numbers by the pattern they make on the phone pad.

Codes. Use dates for telephone or door code numbers, like 1960 or 1845. It works wonders.

Multiplication. When trying to remember your multiplication tables, go to the nearest one you can remember and then add one or double the number. 3x8 is 24, so 6x8 is double that, that is, 48.

Comparing numbers. When visually comparing numbers, you don't always see differences. When you need to compare two large numbers, put one in your calculator's memory and then subtract the other number. The resulting zero answer assures you the numbers are the same.

How many days in the month?Sometimes using this elementary school trick for remembering everyday things such as 'Thirty days hath September, April, June and November; all the rest have thirty-one, except for February which has twenty-eight, works very well.

CHAPTER NINE

Confusing "B" and "D"

Which way round is 'b'?Use the name 'Cadbury's' (chocolate) to help remember which way 'b' and 'd' go.

Which way round is 'b'?To know b from d, try picturing the capital letter B and know that the lower-case b is the bottom of the letter, and the d is facing the opposite direction.

'b' and 'd'.A good tip for getting your b's and d's the right way is to use the word 'bed' and picture yourself lying on it. The 'b' is the headboard and the 'd' is the bit that stops your feet hanging off the end.

You will find it is easier to avoid flipping your letters when writing if you print everything in capital letters. So your lower-case letters are simply smaller upper case.

CHAPTER TEN

Spelling and Grammar Tips

Computer programmes.A great programme from www.texthelp.comwhich reads out loud what you have written. It helps you to spot words you have missed out.

Careful. Avoid overeating sugar or sweeteners, as you will find it can affect your reading and spelling. Always try to eat a healthy diet - fruit, vegetables and vitamin supplements each day.

Word processors. If you find you cannot spell a word, type in a smaller one with the same meaning and use the thesaurus to find the word you need.

Fingerspelling. If you have bad spelling and you find that you have a problem with hearing or knowing the sounds of the letters, try using something called 'fingerspelling'. This is where you put a finger up for each sound you hear in the word. It allows you to "see" the sounds and work out what sounds are missing. It also helps improve your spelling at the same time.

Spelling while typing. When you are either writing or typing things on a computer, mentally spell out each word as you type or write it, instead of just thinking the word. That is, as you type the word "computer", literally think in your head "c-o-m-p-u-t-e-r" as you type it. This way, the word is broken down into its component letters, and you don't have to take extra time to ensure that you have spelt it correctly. This works about 90% of the time unless it is a word that is new to you when it comes to the spelling.

Spelling easier on a keyboard. You will find that spelling is easier when you are using a keyboard and computer. Look at the keys which seem to help some people. Sometimes, anxiety about getting the correct spelling ends up confusing people when they write by hand.

Using a dictionary. When using a dictionary, write the alphabet at the bottom of the page, ABCD then you will know the position of the letters without saying the whole alphabet to yourself.

Spell checker. The spell checker is your best friend. Use it always. Write your notes twice so you can read them. Read something out loud so you can understand it. Always spell-check your writing on your email browser before submitting it in, for example, a forum. Then just cut out the email message.

Read your sentences backwards (to find errors in your writing). Leaving off an "s" "es" or "ed" is easier to spot.

Remember grammar rules. Simple rules like when two vowels go walking, the first one does the talking.

CHAPTER ELEVEN

Using Colour While Dyslexic

Code colouring. Colour code everything. If you need to organise your computer disks, colour code them by the project or by the class they belong. Make labels with the colour and name and place them on the disk, whether it is a CD or zip or floppy. This helps to remember where things are and saves time looking through every disk.

Highlighters. When reading books, read with several highlighters close by. That way, when one 'disappears' you can continue. Almost every book you own should be 'highlighted' to some degree.

Coloured paper. If you only have a mild form of dyslexia, but enough to make life difficult, using coloured sheets of paper will help you to read effortlessly.

Red and blue. If you have major left-right issues and you are ambidextrous, which makes life all the more confusing, wear a Red sock on your right foot and a blue one on your left. When a direction is addressed this way, it will be easier for you to know which is left and which is right.

Coloured pens. When you study, use different coloured pens to focus your attention to the critical points that you need to know.

Use a coloured report cover. Use themover pages in a book. You can use blue, and therefore the words are black, and the background is blue. It can be beneficial when you read. If you are experiencing glare or fuzzy words without your blue transparent plastic cover, you may have Scotopic Sensitivity Syndrome. You may need tinted lenses.

CHAPTER TWELVE

Tips at Work or School

Managing tasks. Put all your personal and work tasks on one sheet of paper. From there, grab a notebook and assign your tasks to specific days of the week, using one piece of paper for each day of the week. Also, assign your tasks a time. When you are done, put the remaining tasks on a single page. These will be your long-term tasks. As you complete tasks during the day, cross them off or re-organise them. The ones that you did not complete, roll them over to another day.

You can also insert birthdays and reminders. An update each day takes about 5 - 10 minutes. When you re-do your plan for the next week, which is usually over the weekend, it takes about 40 - 50 minutes. If you are a visual person who learns best when writing things down, this will work for you. It has worked for many people. One key benefit is that you will feel confident because your tasks are managed, and you have it all captured on paper so that you won't forget things.

Finding a quiet place. When you need a peaceful setting and a quick outline to get your thoughts straight, find a calm place to relax while doing this. Don't worry about spelling on the first draft, just the quality of what you are trying to convey. Your creative side soars using this method. If you run out of ideas, try brainstorming aloud. Reversing the order of things confuses some people so avoid that if you are one of them. To conquer this problem, take it in steps by drawing pictures and talking to yourself. A quiet place is needed to concentrate.

Mark up all the key points. In school, you can keep your books and circle or mark up all key points when reading. Just before each test, you can just read the key or circled points. This method works very well and makes learning easier. However, the books will be in bad condition if you use this method.

Grading tests on content. In school, always ask your teachers to grade on content, not spelling. Most teachers have no problem with this.

Remembering what you read. If you have a hard time remembering what you are reading when you study, try this. When you get to the end of a page in your textbook, write down everything you can remember before moving on. It takes some time but helps in the long run.

Get the lighting right. Some people have found that they can read better if the lighting is right. Bright light tends to slow down the reading of some people. Soft, white light helps focus. Just make sure you are not sleepy.

Too much information. If you are a higher institution student, when under pressure, you will be tempted to gather too much information, and that will make you unable to focus. So try to take a long walk outside or go to a library and pull your thoughts back together. Frequently use an outline of each class for what you want to do, that allows you to focus in a logical order. If you don't understand what you are reading, if your biggest problem is comprehension, the outline helps break the lesson into parts to create a smaller area to focus on.

Before academic work. Just before undertaking academic work, go for a walk, or preferably a run, to get the blood circulating. After the exercise, you will be buzzing and will be far more receptive to learning.

Taking tests. When taking tests, if they are multiple-choice tests, try to make each possible answer a true or false question. It helps to eliminate more choices.

Forhigher institutions examinations, ask the tutor to put three lines of blank spaces between each question on the paper. It will still hard, but at least you can see where one question ends, and the next one starts.

Tutors. Ask a tutor you may haveto print, rather than write, the important words on the board in lectures. This helps a lot with note-taking.

Work manuals. Read manuals on to a tape recorder. Then you can play them back as many times as you like and it sticks in your head.

Planning study time. As a student, you will find planning your time hard work. You will make a plan of all the time slots in a normal day, then colour all the used time in red, and fill the blank slots in green. This helps you visualise the time available for study and other life responsibilities.

Videos and study. If you have great difficulty in reading, so when an assignment from school is given, go to the library and find videos with the subject you need to study. You will find reading much more comfortable once you know the basics. Remember, the brain typically processes twenty minutes of information then shuts off.

MISCELLANEOUS TIPS

Keeping appointments. If you have trouble telling the time and keeping appointments, use the 24-hour time format, so you don't confuse morning with evening appointments. If you have appointment months ahead, always write the date in full, with the year too, if necessary.

Problem with 'scanning'. Some people have a severe problem with "scanning" either for a product on a store shelf or some landmark that someone gave them with directions to where they are going. Some people's most hated nightmare is losing someone in a crowd in a mall or other public place. You will find that letting people know the kind of clarification that you need is the best way.

Using a cash register. If you have worked in a store using a cash register when counting money, try saying aloud the amount, then count to yourself two times the amount going back, then again out loud to the customer.

Giving directions. If you get lost easily, and reading a map is hard for you, and you don't know if you are going north or south, make written directions like 'Go left on X Street', and never let people tell you 'Go along, or up, or down'. Instead, you might like it if they write 'Go to Mary Street' and then say 'It's one past John Street, and if you see Rob Street, turn around.' Also, you may need a full set of instructions to make it home again.

Self-adhesive address labels. Always carry lots of small self-adhesive address labels. It saves time and prevents you from handing out scribbled, difficult-to-read notes. This can happen if you get flustered trying to hurry as people are waiting. Instead of signing your name on forms, use these and have plenty for copies. They are also useful for providing a 'return address' on parcels and for handing out, instead of laboriously writing down your address. It is very cheap to buy heaps of them, and people seem to respond well to receiving them.

Conclusion

We hope the numerous tips and tricks and other resources we have outlined for you will help you in your quest to overcome Adult Dyslexia. We are more than confident that you will succeed and find yourself enjoying life more than before. We would also like to state that not all the tips and tricks may work for everyone. As we have mentioned previously, there is no typical case of dyslexia.

That being said, be sure to try out all of them to see what works for you and what doesn't. We know you will find several them more than helpful for you in your daily life and activities.